Diabetes Diet

Healthy Nutritious Diabetes Recipes to Control & Reverse Type 1 & 2 Diabetes

Table of Contents

Introduction

Chapter 1 - Breakfast

Chapter 2 - Appetizers

Chapter 3 - Main Meals

Chapter 4 - Snacks

Chapter 5 - Desserts

Chapter 6 - Smoothies

Conclusion

Introduction

It is overwhelming and often frightening if you are diagnosed with diabetes, particularly when it comes to maintaining a diet plan. Remember, you can still live a healthy, happy life, even if you are diagnosed with diabetes. You just have to follow the right diet, which is the basis of successful management of diabetes. The guild will show you that diabetic recipes can be both nutritious and exciting and will keep you satisfied, alert and ready for any challenges that life throws at you.

The book will show you how you can enjoy your favorite dishes with a few tweaks. This cookbook contains delicious, tasty recipes that provide healthy, high energy meals covering breakfasts, appetizers, main meals, snacks, desserts and even smoothies. The recipes in this book will help make your mealtimes interesting and healthy and improve blood glucose, blood pressure, cholesterol numbers and help control diabetes.

☐ **Copyright 2016 by Lifesytledawn - All rights reserved.**

Chapter 1 - Breakfast

Asparagus and Cheese Omelet

Ingredients for 1 serving

1/2 teaspoon olive oil

- Nonstick cooking spray
- 3 egg whites
- 3 -5 thin spears asparagus
- 1 tablespoon red sweet pepper slivers
- 1-ounce spreadable cheese wedge, cut up (any flavor, individually foil-wrapped)
- 1/8 teaspoon freshly ground black pepper
- 1 teaspoon fresh parsley (snipped)

Method

1. With cooking spray, lightly coat an unheated large nonstick skillet. Add asparagus to skillet and pan-roast over medium-high heat until browned and crisp-tender, about 7 minutes, turn occasionally. Cover the pan with foil and set aside.
2. Combine egg whites and pepper in a medium bowl and beat with a fork until combined but not frothy. Heat oil over medium-high heat in an 8-inch nonstick skillet. Add egg whites to skillet and lower the heat to medium. Once the eggs start to set, gently lift edges of set egg white with a heatproof silicone spatula and tilt pan to allow liquid egg white to run under the set egg. Continue to cook until egg is set but still shiny.

3. Arrange the asparagus spears on half of the egg in the skillet and top evenly with cheese. Now fold the unfilled half of the egg over the cheese and asparagus.

4. Gently place the omelet onto a serving plate. Sprinkle omelet with parsley and red sweet pepper slivers.

5. Serve.

Nutrition Information

- Calories 116 kcal
- Cholesterol 10mg
- Carbs 4g
- Fat 5g
- Sodium 427mg

Buckwheat Flour and Blueberry Pancake

Ingredients for 6 servings

- 1 egg, slightly beaten
- 3/4 cup fresh or frozen blueberries, thawed
- 1/2 cup buckwheat flour
- 1/4 teaspoon salt
- 1 tablespoon sugar
- 1/4 teaspoon vanilla
- 1/4 teaspoon baking soda
- 1 1/4 cups buttermilk or sour milk
- 1/2 teaspoon baking powder
- 1/2 cup whole wheat flour
- 1 tablespoon cooking oil

Method

1. In a medium bowl, stir together whole wheat flour, buckwheat flour, baking soda, baking powder, sugar, and salt. In the center of the flour mixture, make a well and set aside.

2. Beat egg slightly in a small bowl; stir in vanilla, oil, and buttermilk. Add buttermilk-oil mixture to the flour mixture, all at once. Stir so the mixture is just combined but still slightly lumpy. Stir in the blueberries.

3. Heat a heavy skillet over medium heat and pour ¼ cup batter onto hot skillet for each pancake. With a spatula, spread the batter into a circle that is about 4 inches in diameter.

4. Cook over medium heat for 1 to 2 minutes per side or until pancakes are brown.

5. Serve.

Nutrition Information

- Calories 132 kcal
- Cholesterol 2mg
- Carbs   22g
- Fat   3g
- Sodium 244mg

Scrambled Eggs with Sausage

Ingredients for 2 servings

- 2 eggs
- 2 tablespoons finely shredded reduced-fat cheddar cheese
- 1 whole grain English muffin, halved and toasted
- 1 ounce cooked turkey sausage, sliced
- 1/4 cup cherry tomatoes, quartered
- 2 tablespoons reduced-sodium chicken broth
- Pinch ground black pepper
- Nonstick cooking spray

Method

1. Coat a large nonstick skillet with cooking spray and preheat skillet over medium heat.
2. In a medium bowl, whisk together eggs, black pepper, and broth and then stir in sliced sausage.
3. Into the hot skillet, pour the egg mixture. Cook over medium heat until mixture begins to set on the bottom and around edges, avoid stirring.
4. With a spatula, lift and fold the partially cooked egg mixture so the uncooked portion drops onto the skillet. Continue to cook over medium heat until almost set; add cheese and tomatoes. Cook until egg mixture is cooked through but still glossy and moist, about 1 minute more.
5. Serve over toasted English muffin halves.

Nutrition Information

- Calories 198 kcal
- Cholesterol 231mg
- Carbs   16g
- Fat   9g
- Sodium 524mg

Broccoli and Tomato Frittata

Ingredients for 4 servings

- 1 teaspoon olive oil
- 1/4 cup feta cheese
- 2 tablespoons finely chopped shallots
- 1/4 teaspoon ground black pepper
- 1 1/4 cups cherry tomatoes, quartered
- 6 egg whites
- 2 cups small broccoli florets
- 3 eggs
- 1/4 teaspoon salt

Method

1. Preheat the broiler.
2. In a medium bowl, whisk together eggs, egg whites, salt, and pepper. Stir in cheese and set aside.
3. In a large broiler-proof skillet, cook shallots and broccoli in hot oil over medium heat until tender, about 8 to 10 minutes, stir occasionally.
4. Pour the egg mixture over the shallots-broccoli mixture in skillet and cook over medium-low heat. Once the mixture starts to set, with a spatula, lift the egg mixture around the edge of the skillet so uncooked portion drops onto the skillet. Continue to cook and lift the edges until egg mixture is almost set, but the surface will be moist. Now arrange the tomatoes on top of egg mixture.
5. Broil 4 to 5 inches from the heat until center is set, about 5 minutes. Allow to cool for 5 minutes before serving.

6. Cut into four wedges and serve.

Nutrition Information

- Calories 134 kcal
- Cholesterol 161mg
- Carbs 7g
- Fat 6g
- Sodium 416mg

Chapter 2 - Appetizers

Sushi Roll

Ingredients for 8 servings

- 4 sheets nori seaweed sheets
- 1/2 cucumber, peeled, cut into small strips
- 1/2-pound imitation crabmeat, flaked
- 3 tablespoons white sugar
- 1 avocado
- 2 tablespoons pickled ginger
- 3 tablespoons rice vinegar
- 2/3 cup uncooked short-grain white rice
- 1 1/2 teaspoons salt

Method

1. Bring 1 1/3 cups water to a boil in a medium saucepan. Add rice, stir and reduce heat. Cover the pan and simmer for 20 minutes. In a small bowl, mix the sugar, rice vinegar, and salt. Blend the mixture into the rice.

2. Preheat the oven to 300F. Heat nori on a medium baking sheet in the preheated oven until warm, about 1 or 2 minutes.

3. On a bamboo sushi mat, center one sheet nori. With wet hands, spread a thin layer of rice on the sheet of nori, then press into a thin layer. In a line down the center of the rice, arrange ¼ of the cucumber, avocado, ginger, and imitation crabmeat. Lift the end of the mat and gently roll it over the ingredients. Press gently and roll it

forward to make a complete roll. Repeat the process with the remaining ingredients.

4. With a wet, sharp knife, cut each roll into 4 to 6 slices.

Nutrition Information

- Calories 152 kcal
- Cholesterol 6mg
- Carbs 25.8g
- Fat 3.9g
- Sodium 703mg

Pineapple Salsa

Ingredients for 8 servings

- 1 (15 ounces) can black beans, drained and rinsed
- 1/2 cup diced red bell pepper
- 1 cup frozen corn kernels, thawed
- 2 green chili peppers, chopped
- 1 cup finely chopped fresh pineapple
- 1/4 cup chopped fresh cilantro
- 1/2 cup diced green bell pepper
- 1/4 cup orange juice
- 1/4 cup chopped onions
- 1/2 teaspoon ground cumin
- Salt and pepper to taste

Method

1. In a large bowl, toss together red bell pepper, pineapple, green bell pepper, black beans, corn, green chili peppers, onions, cilantro and orange juice. Season with salt, pepper, and cumin.
2. Cover and chill in the refrigerator until serving.

Nutrition Information

- Calories 95 kcal
- Cholesterol 0mg
- Carbs   19.3g

- Fat   0.5g
- Sodium 207mg

Fried Plantains

Ingredients for 2 servings

- 1 green plantain
- 5 tablespoons oil for frying
- 3 cups cold water
- Salt to taste

Method

1. Peel and cut the plantain into 1-inch chunks.
2. In a large skillet, heat the oil. Add the plantains in the oil and fry on both sides. About 3 ½ minutes per side.
3. Remove the plantains from the pan. Place a plate over the fried plantains and flatten them by pressing down.
4. Dip the flattened plantains in the water and return to the hot oil and fry for another 1 minute, per side.
5. Salt to taste and serve.

Nutrition Information

- Calories 136 kcal
- Cholesterol 0mg
- Carbs   28.5g
- Fat   3.3g
- Sodium 14mg

Grilled Bacon Wrapped New Potatoes

Ingredients for 15 servings

- 1 (1 ounce) package ranch dressing mix
- 15 small new potatoes
- 15 toothpicks
- 5 slices bacon, cut into thirds

Method

1. Preheat the outdoor grill for low heat and then lightly oil the grate.
2. With a piece of bacon, wrap each potato and secure with a toothpick. Sprinkle the potatoes with ranch dressing mix.
3. Place the potatoes on the grill, turn them several times to cook the bacon on all sides. Cook for about 20 to 25 minutes or until the bacon is nice and crispy.

Nutrition Information

- Calories 92 kcal
- Cholesterol 3mg
- Carbs 17g
- Fat 1.4g
- Sodium 207mg

Chapter 3 - Main Meals

Red Lentil Curry

Ingredients for 8 servings

- 1 teaspoon salt
- 1 large onion, diced
- 1 teaspoon minced garlic
- 1 tablespoon vegetable oil
- 1 teaspoon white sugar
- 1 teaspoon chili powder
- 1 (14.25 ounce) can tomato puree
- 1 teaspoon ground cumin
- 1 teaspoon minced fresh ginger
- 2 tablespoons curry paste
- 1 tablespoon curry powder
- 2 cups red lentils
- 1 teaspoon ground turmeric

Method

1. In cold water, wash the lentils until the water runs clear. In a pot, put the lentils and add enough water to cover and bring to a boil. Reduce heat to medium-low, cover with a lid and cook until tender, about 15 to 20 minutes, add water during cooking to keep the lentils moist. Drain.

2. In a large skillet, heat vegetable oil over medium heat. Add onions and cook and stir until caramelized, about 20 minutes.

3. In a large bowl, mix curry powder, curry paste, cumin, turmeric, sugar, garlic, chili powder, ginger, and salt together. Stir into the onions and increase the heat to high and cook until fragrant, about 1 to 2 minutes, stir constantly.

4. Stir in the tomato puree, remove the skillet from the heat and stir into the lentils.

Nutrition Information

- Calories 192 kcal
- Cholesterol 0mg
- Carbs 32.5g
- Fat 2.6g
- Sodium 572mg

BBQ Chicken Salad

Ingredients for 4 servings

- 1/4 cup barbecue sauce
- 1/2 red onion, diced
- 4 stalks celery, chopped
- 1 (8.75 ounces) can sweet corn, drained
- 2 tablespoons fat-free mayonnaise
- 1 large red bell pepper, diced
- 2 skinless, boneless chicken breast halves

Method

1. Preheat grill for high heat and lightly oil grate.
2. Grill chicken until juices run clear, about 10 minutes on each side. Remove from the heat, cool and cube.
3. In a large bowl, toss together the chicken, celery, onion, red bell pepper, and corn.
4. In a small bowl, mix together the mayonnaise and barbecue sauce. Pour over the veggies and chicken. Stir.
5. Chill until ready to serve.

Nutrition Information

- Calories 168 kcal
- Cholesterol 34mg
- Carbs 23.6g
- Fat 2.2g
- Sodium 473mg

Pasta with Tomato Sauce

Ingredients for 8 servings

- 1/2 cup Italian dressing
- 1 (16 ounces) package dry penne pasta
- 8 Roma (plum) tomatoes, diced
- 1/4 cup grated Parmesan cheese
- 1/4 cup finely chopped fresh basil
- 1/4 cup diced red onion

Method

1. Fill a large pot with lightly salted water and bring to a boil. Add the penne pasta in the pot and cook until al dente, about 10 minutes. Drain.
2. In a large bowl, toss the cooked pasta with the Italian dressing, tomatoes, red onion, basil and Parmesan cheese.
3. Serve.

Nutrition Information

- Calories 257 kcal
- Cholesterol 3mg
- Carbs   46.9g
- Fat   3.1g
- Sodium 248mg

BBQ Chicken Pizza

Ingredients for 8 servings

- ¼ cup sugar-free apricot preserves
- 1 (12-inch) pre-packaged whole wheat Italian pizza crust
- ¼ teaspoon ground black pepper
- ½ medium red onion, thinly sliced
- ½ teaspoon hot sauce
- ½ pound boneless, skinless chicken breast
- ¼ cup barbecue sauce
- ½ cup reduced-fat shredded Italian Style cheese
- ¼ teaspoon salt (optional)
- ½ teaspoon dried oregano
- Cooking spray

Method

1. Preheat the oven to 375 F and spray a baking sheet with cooking spray.
2. Season the chicken with pepper and salt (optional) on both sides.
3. Place the chicken on the baking sheet and bake until the juices run clear, about 25 minutes. Remove the chicken from oven and chop into bite size pieces.
4. In a small saucepan, combine the barbecue sauce, sugar-free apricot preserves, and hot sauce. Bring to a boil.

5. Coat the pizza crust with the sauce, top with cooked chicken, sliced onion, and Italian Style cheese. Sprinkle dried oregano over the cheese.

6. Bake the pizza until the cheese is melted and bubbly, about 20-25 minutes.

7. Slice and serve.

Nutrition Information

- Calories 155 kcal
- Cholesterol 20mg
- Carbs   22g
- Fat   3.5g
- Sodium 315mg

Tuna Salad with Chickpeas

Ingredients for 7 servings

- 1 cup canned garbanzo (chickpeas) beans, rinsed and drained
- Ground black pepper ¼ tsp
- 1/2 large red pepper, diced
- 2 medium celery stalks, diced
- Flavor fresh chunk tuna pouches 26.4-ounce, in water
- 1/2 lemon, juiced
- ¼ cup onion, finely diced
- ¼ cup light mayonnaise
- 3 tbsp fat-free plain yogurt

Method

1. In a small bowl, whisk together mayonnaise, lemon juice, and yogurt.
2. Combine the remaining ingredients in a medium bowl. Pour mayonnaise-yogurt mixture over tuna and mix well.
3. Serve tuna salad on your choice of whole-wheat bread and lettuce.

Nutrition Information

- Calories 125 kcal
- Cholesterol 25mg
- Carbs   10g
- Fat   3g

- Sodium 335mg

Chipotle Chilli Salmon

Ingredients for 8 servings

- 1 tbsp lime juice
- 2 tsp coarse salt
- 1 2-lb side of salmon, skin removed
- 1 tbsp light brown sugar
- 1 tbsp olive or canola oil
- 4 chipotle chilli peppers in adobo
- 1 tsp oregano

Method

1. Except salmon, place all ingredients in a blender and puree ingredients together until smooth.
2. Now rub the mixture over the surface of the salmon. On a baking dish, place the salmon and marinate for 20 minutes.
3. Preheat the grill to medium-high. Cook the salmon under direct heat until cook through, about 5-6 minutes on each side.
4. Cool and serve.

Nutrition Information

- Calories 225 kcal
- Cholesterol 80mg
- Carbs   2g
- Fat   2g

- Sodium 435mg

Turkey and Veggie Chili

Ingredients for 8 servings

- 16 ozs lean ground turkey
- 1 small onion, diced
- 1 medium zucchini (6 ounces), diced
- 2 medium carrots, diced
- 1 (15.8 ozs) can great Northern beans, rinsed and drained
- 1 (14.5 ozs) can, no-salt-added diced tomatoes
- 1 clove garlic, minced
- 1 tbsp chili powder
- 1 (28 ozs) can, no-salt-added crushed tomatoes
- 1/2 tsp ground black pepper
- 1 tsp cumin
- 1 (15.25 oz) can no-salt-added kidney beans, rinsed and drained
- 1 tsp garlic powder
- Cooking spray

Method

1. Spray a large pot with cooking spray. Add the carrots, zucchini, and onions, and sauté over medium-high heat until the onions turn clear, about 3-4 minutes. Add the garlic and sauté for another 30 seconds.
2. Add the ground turkey and cook until brown. Now add the remaining ingredients; mix well and bring the

mixture to a boil. Reduce the heat and simmer the mixture for 15 to 20 minutes.

3. Serve.

Nutrition Information

- Calories 235 kcal
- Cholesterol 45mg
- Carbs 27g
- Fat 5g
- Sodium 170mg

BBQ Chicken Burgers

Ingredients for 5 servings

- ¼ teaspoon ground black pepper
- ¼ cup sugar-free barbecue sauce
- 2 teaspoons salt-free steak seasoning
- 1 egg
- ¼ cup oatmeal
- 5 pieces Bibb lettuce
- 16 ounces ground chicken
- 1 tomato, sliced into 5 slices
- 5 small whole wheat hamburger buns (about 1.5 ounces each)
- ¼ teaspoon salt (optional)

Method

1. Preheat the indoor or outdoor grill.
2. In a medium bowl, combine the egg, ground chicken, steak seasoning, oatmeal, salt (optional), and pepper. Mix well.
3. Using your hands, divide the meat mixture into five equal portions and create patties.
4. Grill the patties on one side for about 4 to 5 minutes. Flip the patties and brush the top of each patty with 2 tablespoons of barbecue sauce. Grill the patties for 4 to 5 minutes and flip them again. Now brush the other side with the remaining barbecue sauce. Grill until the patties are cooked through, another 2 to 3 minutes. The internal temperature of the patties should reach 165F.

5. Open one hamburger bun, place the patty on the bottom half of the bun, and top with 1 slice of tomato and 1-piece lettuce. Close the bun. Repeat with the remaining 4 buns.

6. Serve.

Nutrition Information

- Calories 275 kcal
- Cholesterol 105mg
- Carbs   27g
- Fat   10g
- Sodium 240mg

Chapter 4 - Snacks

Parsnip Zucchini and Sweet Potato Chips with Yogurt Dip

Ingredients for 4 servings

- 1/3 cup skim milk
- 1 medium sweet potato, peeled
- 2 tablespoons ranch dressing powder mix
- 1/2 cup non-fat plain Greek yogurt
- 1 medium parsnip
- 1 medium zucchini
- 1 teaspoon salt (optional)

Method

1. Preheat the oven to 200 F. Coast 3 baking sheets with cooking spray.
2. With a mandolin, slice sweet potato, parsnip, and zucchini into 1/8-inch-thick round slices.
3. Line the first baking sheet with parsnips in a single layer, second with sweet potato slices and third with zucchini slices. Spray the slices with cooking spray and season with salt.
4. Bake for 30 to 60 minutes or until the vegetables are crisp and dry; rotate the baking sheets.
5. While the vegetables are in the oven, in a bowl, whisk together the yogurt, milk and ranch powder. Keep in the refrigerator until needed.
6. Cool, the vegetable chips and serve with the dip.

Nutrition Information (Serving size: ½ cup chips and ¼ cup dip)

- Calories 90 kcal
- Carbs 17g
- Fat 0.0g
- Protein 5g

Sweet and Savory Baked Apples

Ingredients for 6 servings

- 2 Honey Crisp Apples (medium size), peeled, seeded and diced
- 6 tbsp Slivered Almonds
- 6 Five-ounce Ramekins
- 6 each light spreadable cheese wedges
- 2 tbsp no-trans-fat margarine
- 2 tbsp Splenda Brown Sugar
- 2 Granny Smith Apples (medium size), peeled, seeded and diced
- 1/8 tsp. Ground Nutmeg
- Cooking Spray
- ¼ tsp. salt (optional)

Method

1. Preheat the oven to 350F.
2. Coat each ramekin with cooking spray and place on a baking sheet.
3. In a medium mixing bowl, combine margarine, apples, Splenda brown sugar, nutmeg, and salt. Combine well.
4. Fill each ramekin about half full with apples and top with one cheese wedge. Gently press to spread over the apples.
5. Now fill the ramekins with the remaining apples.

6. Bake the apples in the oven for 30 minutes. Remove and top each ramekin with one tablespoon of slivered almonds. Place in the oven again to finish baking.

7. Bake another 15 minutes or apples are bubbling and almonds are toasted. Remove from the oven and allow to cool.

8. Serve.

Nutrition Information

- Calories 150 kcal
- Carbs 17g
- Fat 4g
- Protein 8g

Oven-Baked Potato Wedges

Ingredients for 4 servings

- 1 ½ pounds (750 g) large roasting potatoes
- 1 tablespoon olive oil
- Pinch of salt

Method

1. Preheat the oven to 400F and lightly grease a baking tray with 1 teaspoon of the oil.
2. Wash and peel the potatoes, and then cut into ¾ inch thick wedges. Put them in a clean dish towel and pat dry.
3. Spread the wedges on the baking tray and drizzle the wedges with the remaining oil, toss to coat well.
4. Bake until golden brown, about 40 minutes, turn occasionally.
5. Season with salt and serve hot.

Nutrition Information

- Calories 163 kcal
- Carbs 25g
- Fat 5g
- Protein 5g
- Sodium 78mg

Glazed Carrots

Ingredients for 6 servings

- 1 tablespoon honey
- 1 tablespoon butter
- 3 carrots

Method

1. Wash and peel the carrots, then cut into ¼ inch slices on a slight diagonal. Cook in a saucepan of boiling water over medium heat until just tender, about 5 minutes. Drain off the liquid and return the carrots and pan to the stovetop.
2. Add the honey and butter to the pan. Cook over low heat, stirring and tossing until the carrots are well glazed, about 2 minutes.
3. Serve.

Nutrition Information

- Calories 46 kcal
- Carbs 6g
- Fat 3g
- Protein 5g
- Sodium 37mg

Fruit and Nut Energy Squares

Ingredients for 16 squares

- Canola oil spray
- 2 tablespoons pepitas (pumpkin seeds)
- 65 g (2¼ ozs/¼ cup) unsweetened apple purée
- 2 eggs
- 2 tablespoons unsweetened cocoa powder
- 2 tablespoons roasted almonds, chopped
- 50 g (1¾ ozs) dried figs, finely chopped
- 1 tablespoon linseeds (flaxseeds)
- 50 g (1¾ ozs/½ cup) rolled (porridge) oats
- 2 tablespoons roasted hazelnuts, chopped
- 50 g (1¾ oz/½ cup) lupin flour
- 2 tablespoons canola oil
- 100 g (3½ ozs) dried apricots, finely chopped
- 65 g (2¼ ozs/½ cup) oat bran

Method

1. Preheat the oven to 325F and lightly spray an 8-inch square cake tin with canola oil. Then line the sides and base with baking paper, let the paper extend over the sides.

2. In a bowl, put the cocoa, oats, oat bran, flour, figs, apricots, almonds, hazelnuts, linseeds and half the pepitas and mix well.

3. In a small bowl, whisk the eggs, canola oil, and apple puree. Then pour into the dry ingredients and mix until combined.

4. Into the prepared tin, press the fruit and nut mixture and scatter over the remaining pepitas.

5. Bake until the slice is firm, about 25-30 minutes. Cool in the tin for 30 minutes, then bring it out and cut into 16 squares.

Nutrition Information

- Calories 515 kcal
- Carbs 11g
- Fat 1g
- Protein 5g
- Sodium 30mg

Chapter 5 - Desserts

Sweet Potato Pudding

Ingredients for 10 servings

- 1/2 cup (30 g) shaved coconut
- 1 large egg, lightly beaten
- 4 large egg whites, lightly beaten
- 1/2 teaspoon (2 ml) ground ginger
- 2 teaspoons (10 ml) vegetable oil
- 1 tablespoon (15 ml) vegetable oil
- 1/2 teaspoon (2 ml) ground cloves
- 1/2 cup (115 g) firmly packed soft brown sugar
- 1/2 teaspoon (2 ml) ground allspice
- 2 tablespoons (30 ml) orange juice concentrate
- 11/2 cups (375 ml) light evaporated milk
- 2 orange sweet potatoes, about 1 pound (500 g), peeled, grated
- Pinch of salt

Method

1. Preheat the oven to 350F and lightly grease an 8 cup (2 liters) baking dish with the oil.
2. In a large bowl, combine all the ingredients except the coconut. Pour the sweet potato mixture into the baking dish and cover with foil.

3. Bake the pudding for an hour. Top with the coconut and bake until the center is set and the coconut turns golden, another 10 minutes.

Nutrition Information

- Calories 178 kcal
- Carbs   25g
- Fat   6g
- Protein 7g
- Sodium 137mg

Lemon Mousse with Strawberries

Ingredients for 8 servings

- 1 cup (250 g) strawberries, hulled and sliced thickly
- 2 teaspoons (10 ml) finely grated lemon zest
- 1 tablespoon (15 ml) extra light olive oil
- 1/2 cup (125 ml) freshly squeezed lemon juice
- 1 1/3 cups (340 ml) fat-free plain yogurt
- 3/4 cup (165 g) sugar
- 1 large egg
- 2 teaspoons (10 ml) powdered gelatin

Method

1. In a small bowl, put 3 tablespoons cold water. Sprinkle gelatin evenly over the water and let soften for about 5 minutes.
2. In a saucepan, put another 3 tablespoons water, egg, sugar, lemon zest, lemon juice and oil and whisk together until well combined.
3. Place the pan over a low heat and cook until the mixture is hot, about 5 minutes, whisk constantly. Now whisk in the softened gelatin and cook until gelatin has dissolved, whisk constantly.
4. Remove from the heat and transfer the mixture to a bowl. Whisk occasionally and allow to cool. Whisk in the yogurt.
5. Layer lemon mousse and strawberries into eight dessert bowls and place in the fridge to chill until set, about 3 hours.

Nutrition Information

- Calories 148 kcal
- Carbs 26g
- Fat 3g
- Protein 5g
- Sodium 52mg

Nutmeg Grape Jelly

Ingredients for 4 servings

- 2 tablespoons (30 ml) superfine sugar
- 1 cup (250 ml) red grape juice
- Greek-style yogurt, to serve
- 1/2 small orange
- 2 teaspoons (10 ml) powdered gelatin
- 1 cup (250 ml) red wine
- 2 star anise
- 1 cup (250 g) seedless red or black grapes
- Pinch of freshly grated nutmeg, to serve

Method

1. Cut the grapes in half if large or leave the grapes whole if they are small. Divide among four large glass tumblers and keep them in the fridge to chill.

2. Start to make the jelly. From the orange half, thinly slice a long strip of zest, squeeze the juice from the orange and set aside. Place the zest in a saucepan with the star anise and wine. Gently heat until almost boiling, lower the heat, cover the pan and simmer for 10 minutes. Remove the pan from the heat, add the sugar, then stir and dissolve.

3. Strain the sweetened wine into a bowl and sprinkle the gelatin over the surface and stir gently until dissolved. Add the grape juice and the reserved orange juice and set aside to cool until the liquid is lukewarm, about 5 minutes.

4. Bring out the grape glasses, pour the jelly mixture over the grapes and set aside until completely cool. Then place in the fridge until set, about 4 hours.

5. Top with yogurt and sprinkled with nutmeg and serve.

Nutrition Information

- Calories 176 kcal
- Carbs 29g
- Fat 1g
- Protein 3g
- Sodium 25mg

Lemon Yogurt Blueberry Parfait

Ingredients for 4 servings

- 1 tablespoon vanilla
- 2 small lemons, zested and juiced
- ¼ cup Splenda
- 1 cup fresh blueberries
- 32 ozs nonfat, plain Greek yogurt
- ¼ cup sliced almonds

Method

1. In a mixing bowl, whisk together lemon juice, lemon zest, yogurt, and Splenda.
2. To a parfait glass, add ½ cup yogurt and top with ¼ cup blueberries. Then add another ½ cup of yogurt. Sprinkle 1 tablespoon sliced almond on top.
3. Repeat the process with the other three parfait glasses.
4. Serve immediately or keep in the refrigerator.

Nutrition Information

- Calories 200 kcal
- Carbs 19g
- Fat 3.5g
- Protein 25g

Chapter 6 - Smoothies

Blueberry Cherry and Banana Smoothies

Ingredients for 4 servings

- Fresh or frozen blueberries - 1/2 cup, unsweetened
- 1 small banana, peeled
- Blueberry-flavored Greek nonfat yogurt (1 6 - ounce carton)
- 1 cup unsweetened vanilla-flavored almond milk
- Frozen unsweetened sour cherries (1 1/2 cups)

Method

1. Combine milk, cherries, yogurt, blueberries and banana in a blender. Cover and pour into glasses to serve.

Nutrition Information

- Calories 104 Kcal
- Carbs 20g
- Fat 1g
- Protein 5g
- Sodium 62mg

Green Tea Chia Seeds and Mango Smoothies

Ingredients for 4 servings

- 2 cups frozen mango chunks
- 1 cup sliced carrots or packaged peeled baby carrots
- 4 green tea bags
- 1 teaspoon honey
- 1 tablespoon Chia seeds
- 1-inch fresh ginger, thinly sliced
- 3 cups water

Method

1. In a small saucepan, bring water to boil and then add carrots, cover and cook until very tender, about 10 to 15 minutes. Add ginger slices for the last 2 minutes of cooking. Remove the pan from the heat. Add tea bags, cover and steep for 4 minutes.
2. Remove ginger slices and tea bags, squeeze out all the tea. Set pan on a hot pad in the refrigerator for about 10 minutes. In a blender, add carrot mixture, Chia, honey, and mango. Cover and blend until smooth.
3. Pour into glasses and serve.

Nutrition Information

- Calories 69 Kcal
- Carbs   17g
- Fiber   2g
- Protein   1g

- Sodium 27mg

Apricot Nectar and Peaches Smoothies

Makes 6 servings

- 2 medium peaches, peeled, pitted, and sliced
- 1 1/2 cups crushed ice
- 1 tablespoon lemon juice or lime juice
- 15 1/2 - ounce can apricot nectar, chilled
- 1 1/2 cups carbonated water, chilled

Method

1. In a blender, combine peaches, apricot nectar, lemon or lime juice and crushed ice. Cover and blend until smooth.
2. Pour fruit mixtures into tall glasses and top with carbonated water.
3. Serve.

Nutrition Information

- Calories 40 Kcal
- Carbs 10g
- Fiber 1g
- Sodium 14mg

Chocolate and Banana Smoothies

Ingredients for 4 servings

- 3 tablespoons unsweetened cocoa powder
- 2 tablespoons honey
- 2 cups fat-free milk
- 1 banana, sliced and frozen
- 1 teaspoon vanilla

Method

1. In a blender, combine banana, milk, honey, cocoa powder, and vanilla.
2. Cover and blend until smooth and frothy.
3. Serve.

Nutrition Information

- Calories 122 Kcal
- Carbs   23g
- Fat   1g
- Fiber   1g
- Sodium 65mg

Strawberry Raspberry and Blueberry Smoothies

Ingredients for 4 servings

- 1 cup pomegranate juice
- 3 tablespoons sugar-free vanilla flavor protein powder
- 2 cups frozen unsweetened strawberries
- 1 cup fresh blackberries or blueberries
- 1 cup frozen unsweetened raspberries
- 1 cup fresh baby spinach leaves

Method

1. In a blender, combine blueberries, strawberries, raspberries, pomegranate juice, spinach and protein powder.
2. Cover and blend until smooth.
3. Serve.

Nutrition Information

- Calories 118 Kcal
- Carbs 26g
- Fat 1g
- Fiber 5g
- Sodium 37mg

Conclusion

By following guidelines and meal plans, you can still live a healthy life, even if you have developed diabetic conditions.

www.ingramcontent.com/pod-product-compliance
Lightning Source LLC
Chambersburg PA
CBHW06042 1190526
45169CB00002B/998